Maximizing Fertility Through Nutrition: A Guide For Preconception Health

GLEN ROBERT

1

Table of contents

Introduction

Concluding that you want to have a family is a beautiful and transformative event in one's life. As soon as you have made that choice, the last thing you want is to have difficulties in having a child. In the same vein, you want the pregnancy to go as smoothly as possible, and you want the kid to be as healthy as ever. When it comes to the contemporary environment, this involves minimizing your exposure to contaminants, ensuring that you are receiving the proper nourishment, and making your life more organized.

Overconsumption of sugar, junk, processed food, caffeine, and alcohol, indoor, sedentary lifestyles, and weight concerns all lead to lower reproductive health. The capacity to conceive, have a healthy baby and pregnancy, and have a good delivery may all be negatively impacted by being overweight or underweight, according to Dr. Francesca Naish, a fertility specialist.

Problems with fertility are everything but a problem that just affects women. Swisse Wellness Expert Dr. David Cannata is quoted as saying, "It is very important that both parents participate in a preconception health program and that they do so together." It is very well documented that the health of a woman during preconception not only affects the capacity to conceive but is also strongly connected to a good pregnancy and the growth of the kid. The preconceived notions that men have about their health are equally significant.

Cannata says, "Male sperm health is easily influenced by diet and lifestyle and poor health can be a common factor in couples struggling to conceive. Furthermore, male preconception health may also impact early pregnancy development, thus it is crucial for both parents to partake in a health program during preconception.``

Research suggests that people who follow a program of good preconception care have a higher pregnancy success rate, healthier babies, better deliveries, and fewer difficulties in pregnancy. A favorable result is most probable when both parents are active, and stick strictly to guidelines.

In a 1995 UK study of 367 couples by Foresight and Surrey University, 81 percent of previously infertile couples who followed a preconception program, successfully conceived a child. Of all births occurring throughout the two-year study period, there were no miscarriages, perinatal deaths, abnormalities, or newborns referred to critical care. According to the research authors, a typical predicted result for a sample of such size would have been 70 miscarriages and six deformities. In fact, before joining the health program, 38 percent of the participating couples had previously been touched by miscarriage, 11 percent by therapeutic abortion, three percent by stillbirth, 2 percent by deformities, and one percent by SIDS.

Chapter 1

What is preconception health?

Preconception health is your health before pregnancy. Being healthy before pregnancy can help improve your chances of getting pregnant. It also can help prevent pregnancy complications when you do get pregnant. Good preconception health includes getting a preconception checkup and talking to your health care provider about health conditions that can affect your pregnancy. It also includes taking folic acid to help prevent birth defects and making changes in your life that may affect the health of your baby when you do get pregnant.

If you're thinking about getting pregnant, start focusing on your health at least 3 months before you start trying to get pregnant. If you have health conditions that may affect a pregnancy, you may need longer to get your body ready to have a baby.

Preparing for a healthy pregnancy, preconception care, should be the norm and a more actively managed step in primary care. Decades of improvement in the quality of maternity care have greatly reduced the risks associated with pregnancy and childbirth, but improvements in preconception care have lagged behind. The health of women as they enter pregnancy remains a major challenge to maternity services, and two-thirds of maternal deaths in the UK are now in women with pre-existing medical conditions.[1]

Animal and human research show clear links between preconception influences and offspring health extending across two or more generations.2 In the UK and most other countries, preconception health is frequently compromised by maternal and paternal obesity, dietary deficiencies, smoking, excessive alcohol consumption, mental health issues, and recreational drug use, all of which are associated with poorer pregnancy outcomes and frequently rooted in social and economic deprivation.

The rise in obesity among women of reproductive age has been the most pressing 'wake-up call' to improve preconception health. Obesity (body mass index [BMI] ≥30 kg/m2), which affects over one in five (21.6%) pregnant women in the UK,3 is strongly linked to almost all adverse pregnancy and birth outcomes, notably pre-eclampsia, gestational diabetes, and stillbirth, and has lasting consequences for the health of the offspring.4 Unfortunately, attempts to tackle the problem through diet and physical activity interventions starting in pregnancy have had negligible effect on immediate and later outcomes.5,6 Together, these findings call for a new focus on improving health before conception.

Why does preconception health matter for women?

Being as healthy as possible in the months before you try to have a baby has been shown to boost your chances of falling pregnant.

It can also give your baby a better chance of good health throughout their whole life.

Studies have shown that poor health around the time you get pregnant can affect:

- your baby's growth both in your womb and after they are born
- labor and birth

If you want to get pregnant, these simple steps to take before you get pregnant can help you become as healthy and fit as possible:

- be in a healthy weight range
- quit smoking
- take folic acid and iodine supplements
- stop or reduce your alcohol intake
- treat health conditions that could affect your fertility

If you had any complications with a previous pregnancy it's important that you discuss these with your doctor before you try to fall pregnant again.

What is a preconception checkup?

A preconception checkup is a medical checkup you get before pregnancy. It helps your health care provider make sure you're healthy and that your body is ready for pregnancy. The checkup helps your provider treat and sometimes prevent health conditions that may affect your pregnancy. For example, your provider checks to make sure your vaccinations are up to date and gives you any you need before pregnancy.

If you can, get your preconception checkup with the health care provider you want to take care of you when you do get pregnant. You can get a preconception checkup any time. Get one even if you've already had a baby. Your health may have changed since you were last pregnant.

Chapter 2

How Nutrition Impacts Preconception

Adopting a healthy diet is essential prior to conceiving, says Brian Levine, M.D., the practice director at CCRM Fertility Clinic in New York City. "Innumerable studies have demonstrated that foods rich in omega-3 fatty acids, low in sugar, high in antioxidants and lacking in preservatives are directly correlated with better overall general health, but also specifically markedly improve female and male fertility," he says. What's more, diets laden in saturated fats and sugars are linked to higher rates of infertility.

Nutrients play a role in fertility because they may impact ovulation, an essential reproductive function, balance hormones necessary for conception and affect everything from the quality of an embryo to implantation success rates in in-vitro fertilization.

And during pregnancy, a fetus becomes "parasitic," says Dr. Levine, taking nutrients from the expectant person. If you start pregnancy with an inadequate diet, lacking in the essential nutrients your body and your fetus need, you may set yourself up for deficiencies.

"The best way to protect the unborn fetus is to eat and supplement mindfully," says Dr. Levine, adding that lifestyle changes like vomiting alcohol, ceasing smoking, including ample exercise and maintaining a healthy weight are also critical throughout pregnancy.

The most important nutrients to include in your preconception diet

Keeping to a healthy diet is very important for maximizing fertility, but what exactly does a "healthy diet" mean? Although there are more nutrients that play into your fertility and general health than just the ones listed below, the following vitamins and minerals are some of the more vital ones to work into your preconception diet.

Vitamin D

Vitamin D is one of the most important nutrients for female fertility, as it helps regulate your hormones, and ovulation. In fact, one study conducted by researchers at Yale found that 93% of infertile females have Vitamin D deficiencies. Most people get their Vitamin D from the sun, but milk is often fortified with the vitamin, and many multivitamins will also contain some Vitamin D.

Vitamin B6

A member of the B vitamin group, B6 has wonderful fertility benefits, including helping to lengthen the luteal phase, and increase cervical fluid. B6 is also beneficial during early pregnancy as it could help curb nausea. Some of the best food sources of B6 include sunflower seeds, pistachios, and fish.

Iron

Not only does iron help you build healthy new red blood cells, but it also helps boost fertility. Research shows that women who take iron supplements can decrease their risk of ovulatory infertility by about 40%, and it's vital during pregnancy for a baby's development. You may want to consider an iron supplement as you begin your TTC and pregnancy journey, but iron is also found in high quantities in meat, pumpkin seeds, and beans, among others. (Though you should, of course, talk to your healthcare provider before you start taking any supplement.)

Omega-3s
These fatty acids are crucial for helping to regulate your hormones, and therefore your menstrual cycle, and are also very important during pregnancy as babies use it to help them develop their brains. Some individuals choose to take a fish oil supplement for their Omegas, but other sources include fish and eggs. (Though, again, you should talk to your healthcare provider before taking a supplement.)

Folate/folic acid
Folic acid, or folate when it occurs naturally, is vital for DNA synthesis and new cell production, and is linked to better fertility outcomes. It's also important to start taking folic acid before conceiving, as babies use it to help develop their brains within just the first few weeks of pregnancy. Some good sources of folate include citrus fruits, and dark, leafy greens.

Vitamin C
Beyond just protecting your immune system, Vitamin C has lots of specific fertility benefits, like helping to regulate your hormones, and menstrual cycle, most commonly by helping to lengthen the luteal phase. Fruits and vegetables tend to be among the best sources of Vitamin C.

The bottom line
Although it's important to get the recommended amount of certain specific nutrients, it's more important to eat a balanced, healthy diet as a whole - chances are, if you do this, you'll probably get all the good nutrients you need. But if you have questions about whether or not you're getting the nutrients you need in your current diet, or whether or not it's a good idea for you to take a supplement, be sure to talk to your healthcare provider who can answer your questions and provide you with guidance.

Chapter 3

What can you do before you get pregnant to help you have a healthy pregnancy?

Here's what you can do:

- Don't smoke, drink alcohol or take street drugs. All of these can make it harder for you to get pregnant. And they're harmful to your baby when you do get pregnant. Tell your provider if you need help to quit. Also, stay away from secondhand smoke. This is smoke from someone else's cigarettes, cigar or pipe.

- Take prescription drugs exactly as your provider says. Don't abuse prescription drugs. A prescription drug is one your provider says you can take to treat a health condition. You need a prescription (an order from your provider) to get the drug. When you take any medicine, don't take more than your provider says you can take, don't take it with alcohol or other drugs and don't take anyone else's prescription medicine. Make sure any provider who prescribes you medicine knows that you're trying to get pregnant.

- Protect yourself from viruses and infections that may affect pregnancy. These include toxoplasmosis and lymphocytic choriomeningitis (also called LCMV). Toxoplasmosis is an infection you can get from eating undercooked meat or touching cat poop. You can get LCMV from caring for rodents, such as hamsters, mice and guinea pigs. If you have these kinds of pets or a cat, ask someone to care for them and to clean the litter box for you. And make sure any meat you eat is fully cooked.

- Don't use harmful chemicals at home or work. Ask your provider if chemicals you use can affect your chances of getting pregnant or your baby's health when you do get pregnant. Some chemicals can cause birth defects in your baby. If you work with chemicals, talk to your boss about changing job duties before and during pregnancy.

- Reduce your stress. High levels of stress can cause problems during pregnancy, so find ways to manage stress before you get pregnant. Being active, eating healthy and getting plenty of sleep can help you deal with stress. If you're really stressed out, tell your provider. He can help you find a counselor to help you reduce and handle your stress. And get help if you've been abused by your partner. Abuse often gets worse during pregnancy.

Chapter 4

No matter where you are on your fertility journey, there are ways to help optimize your health and improve your pregnancy outcomes. If you are trying to get pregnant and it's taking you longer than you expected, if you have been struggling with fertility issues, or you are just starting your pregnancy journey, I encourage you to not lose hope in your body. There's lots you can do to promote your fertility. One of the most powerful places to start is with your nutrition.

Every woman's path to conception is unique and fertility is very complex. However, despite what you may read or are told, there are many ways in which you can take charge of your fertility. By preparing for conception, you can overcome many fertility issues and improve your chances for a healthy pregnancy.

The foods and nutrients you eat can help reduce inflammation, rebalance hormones, support your immunity, improve detoxification, and nourish your ovaries and uterus. All of which are important factors for fertility, conception, and prenatal health.

What is optimal fertility nutrition?

Eating for optimal fertility focuses on providing your body with the necessary nutrients to support ovulation, pregnancy and a healthy baby. For some, a fertility diet may mean making minor tweaks to the foods and beverages you consume so that you supply your body with the optimal nutrients to support conception and pregnancy.

There has been extensive research showing the powerful connection between nutrition and getting (and staying) pregnant. What we eat directly impacts our fertility, including our menstrual cycle regularity, egg quality, immune health, and the health of your uterine lining. All of which influences your fertility. Ultimately, the research has shown that refining what you eat can have a positive impact on most root causes of fertility issues including PCOS, endometriosis, anovulatory infertility, and more.

The ideal foods for fertility provide your body the support it needs for conception, pregnancy, and for baby's health. By intentionally creating a healthy nutrient status for yourself, you are providing the building blocks for your hormones and your baby.

Chapter 5

Fertility Nutrition Guide: What to eat when trying to get pregnant

The term "fertility diet" was coined after extensive research was completed at the Harvard School of Public Health on the relationship between diet and anovulatory infertility (the lack of ovulation common in PCOS). The study showed that following a fertility diet can influence fertility in healthy women and in women experiencing ovulation issues.

The fertility diet is intended to help women focus on:

Healthy, monounsaturated oils/fats, especially olive oil and avocados, instead of trans fats
Vegetable protein sources like beans, legumes, nuts, and seeds rather than animal protein
Whole grains and low glycemic carbohydrates, and
Organic, high-fat dairy (if well-tolerated)

In addition, I also suggest:

eating organic when possible especially with your proteins, fats and the produce listed on EWG's dirty dozen
avoiding toxins in your foods and associated food prep items, and eating lots and lots of colorful vegetables every day (think about "eating the rainbow")

If you are trying to get pregnant, ask yourself – is my diet packed with foods that will help support my fertility?

Our fertility nutrition guide, along with a good quality prenatal and a few other nutrients, can help optimize your body's functions no matter if you are trying to get pregnant the "old-fashioned way" or are working to conceive through IVF.

Fruits and Vegetables

Diversity is the key to eating fruits and vegetables in the fertility diet. Fill your plate with a rainbow of foods so that you can maximize the minerals, vitamins, and polyphenols that naturally help lower inflammation and control blood sugars. Aim for five to ten servings of fruits and vegetables each day. If you are prone to yeast infections, rashes, or have digestive issues, then limit fruits to 1-2/day and focus more on vegetables, especially leafy greens.

Healthy Fats

Focus on consuming healthy, plant-based fats such as avocados, nuts and seeds (walnuts, pecans, cashews, pumpkin seeds, hemp seeds, flax seeds, sunflower seeds, sesame seeds, pine nuts, etc), and organic, extra virgin olive oil. These fats promote regular ovulation and reduce inflammation in the body. Both of which are important for fertility.

Complex Carbohydrates

For most women, there is no need to cut out carbohydrates altogether. Instead, focus on whole grains and the slow-burning carbohydrates found in foods like quinoa, buckwheat, amaranth, and nut butters. Adding complex carbohydrates to a meal will help keep you fuller longer while also maintaining steady blood sugar levels.

Protein

Diversify your sources of protein. Meat and seafood do not need to be your main sources of protein. Studies have shown that when increasing your intake of plant-based protein by only five percent, your risk of ovulatory disorders can be cut in half. Focus on cold-water fish (wild-caught salmon and trout), plant-based protein (eggs, beans, lentils, nuts, and seeds), and lean meats (chicken and turkey) for protein. If you choose to include red meat in your diet, look for organic, grass-fed, and hormone-free beef. Additionally, pork should be avoided as it can promote inflammation.

I also want to call out a fertility superfood - EGGS!

Eggs are a great source of protein and choline. Choline is an essential nutrient that helps to reduce the occurrence of miscarriage, neural tube defects, and can help improve egg quality. Your body can only produce a small amount of choline and research shows we don't utilize choline well from supplements, so the majority must come from your diet.

Water

Water is the most essential nutrient for our body. Our body relies on water to help with temperature control, lubrication of our tissues and organs, transportation of hormones, removal of wastes, and much more. Grab your water bottle and aim to drink about half of your body weight in ounces of water each day. If you drink caffeine or work out, then add 8 ounces of water for every cup of caffeinated beverage and for every 30 minutes of activity.

Whole, Organic Foods

When possible, focus on eating whole, unprocessed, organic foods. Pesticides and herbicides can act as endocrine disruptors, which can negatively impact your fertility by affecting your (and your growing baby's) hormones and detoxification processes. Some herbicides and pesticides can accumulate more in fat so if possible, buy organic when it comes to fat and proteins (nuts, seeds, meat, fish, oils, etc). Also, become familiar with the Environmental Working Group's clean 15 and dirty dozen food lists to avoid produce that requires more pesticides and herbicides. These lists are updated yearly.

Fertility Nutrition – Foods to Avoid

Fertility nutrition focuses on consuming foods that promote regular ovulation and healthy egg or sperm production. Certain foods can have the opposite effect causing women to make fewer, less healthy eggs. Focus on removing these types of foods or consuming them in moderation.

Trans Fats

Trans fats, found primarily in commercial baked goods, french fries, and animal products increase insulin resistance. Insulin resistance makes it harder for the body to move glucose into the cells causing a build-up of glucose in the body. High levels of glucose can affect regular ovulation. Focus instead on consuming healthy fats (see above).

Caffeine

Avoid or limit caffeine intake from coffee and teas to under 200 milligrams a day. This is the equivalent of one 12 ounce cup of coffee per day. Avoid energy drinks altogether. They are loaded with not only caffeine, but artificial ingredients and food colorings. These have been shown to negatively affect hormones - this especially applies to men and their sperm!

Food Additives and Food Coloring

Many additives or coloring found in commercially produced foods are endocrine disruptors. Endocrine disruptors alter your normal hormone functions and can impact your fertility. Read the labels of the food and beverages you purchase. Look for coloring and additives such as monosodium glutamate (MSG), sodium nitrite, carrageenan, high fructose corn syrup, and aspartame. Also be cautious with "natural flavor" or "artificial flavor" (even in natural or organic products) as these can be code for natural or artificial emulsifiers, solvents, preservatives, or other harmful chemicals that can be harmful to your and your baby's body.

Fish High in Mercury

The reality is that our oceans are becoming more and more toxic from farm and city runoff and commercial dumping of chemicals. These chemicals and toxins, including heavy metals are being found in sea animals and when we eat these animals, we can acquire these chemicals. Mercury and other heavy metals can affect ovulation, conception, and baby's health. I suggest avoiding or minimizing eating large fish that can accumulate metals from eating smaller fish. This includes tuna, swordfish, and any farmed fish. Instead, eat cold-water, wild-caught salmon, cod, sardines, and trout.

Food and Beverages in Plastic

Bisphenol A, also known as BPA and its cousins (BPS and BPF), have been shown to impact both male and female fertility. Bisphenols, commonly found in hard plastics used for food and beverage storage, can accumulate within our body and act as endocrine disruptors, impacting fertility and the success of IVF treatments. Try to use water bottles and food storage containers that are stainless steel or glass. And try to avoid food wrapped in plastic.

A Word of Caution

While the demand for greater nutrients may be higher during pregnancy, parents-to-be should always take safety into consideration. "Just because something is natural doesn't mean it's safe at certain doses," says Dr. Silverberg. "Contact your doctor before introducing any new supplement into your regimen."